The Power of Healthy Habits

Table of Contents

Introduction

I want to thank you and congratulate you for downloading the book, Power of Healthy Habits.

Habits are important to your life because they influence so much about us. They are going to define what habits are considered usual for you, what feelings that you have, the thoughts you think about, and your overall character. This is why bad habits can make someone seem bad; they are acting in that way due to their habits. This does not mean that change is impossible, but it is going to take some conscious efforts to see this change come about.

Creating good habits takes some motivation and hard work. Your body and brain are working against you in order to force you to keep the old habits that you are used to. But when you stick with it and follow the tips in this guidebook, you will find that it is possible to get rid of all your bad habits and exchange them for the good ones that you truly deserve.

Everyone has some bad habits that they wish they could get rid of. They may eat more food than they want, not exercise enough, smoke, drink, or do something else that has become a habit they are a bit ashamed of. Others wish they were able to make the changes needed in order to create some good habits that they could be proud of. With the help of this guidebook, you will find that it is easier to take care of your bad habits while implementing some good habits, and get to where you want to get in the future.

When you want things to change it begins with yourself. This book gives you great ideas for taking better care of yourself by creating good and highly effective habits, because after all you are the only you that you have. You need to consider investing in yourself— your care, your happiness, and your health— before you can invest in other things.

Thanks again for downloading this book, I hope you enjoy it!

Chapter 1 The Mindset

Improving your life is a common shared goal that most people continually work toward over the course of their life. While a lot of these people manage to successfully achieve these desired improvements, the vast majority seems to fail. What is the reason? Do those who are successful possess some kind of special ability that enables them to achieve their goal? Or is it a matter of persistence and dedication? Fortunately, the answer is not as difficult as you might think. It all comes down to a good mindset and the creation of good, highly effective habits.

It is said that it takes approximately thirty days for the average person to successfully change or create a new habit. The reason for this is because most of us don't fully commit our minds to achieving the new goal. We often tend to focus on the negatives such as the time and effort that it will take us to accomplish the task rather than the positive benefits that the new habit will bring. In order to be successful in creating any new habit you have to learn to think positive and foresee a positive future. This will ultimately enable you to achieve anything you desire.

Any improvement of your life comes down to a single thought. That is because a thought creates a signal and draws in thoughts that are similar in tone. For those who pay attention to the tone and focus on those that give them joy and positive emotions, it is easier to move toward success. Therefore, your choice to focus on positive thoughts means other positive thoughts will follow.

When you set your mindset to one full of positive thoughts, you also naturally impact other aspects of your life. Those aspects are usually important ones such as financial stability and your overall satisfaction. When you create good habits, you enrich your life in a natural progression.

Chapter 2 Why Are Habits Important?

First we make our habits, then our habits make us. In fact, it would be very confusing to the brain to try and go through life without some habits. These habits are going to make some of your routine activities more automatic so that your mind is able to be free for other activities. For example, brushing your teeth in the morning does not require a lot of thinking and so you are able to do it while getting dressed or making some breakfast. This is because brushing your teeth is so habitual that you don't need to think about.

Basically, the habits in your life are going to be important because they limit the sensory stimuli that your brain needs to deal with and effectively simplifies your life. They save you energy and don't require a ton of mental or physical strength.

When you have good habits, you are able to use those habits in order to be efficient, keep things in order, and to create a routine. They can also keep your body healthy and happy, such as when you start exercising. On the other hand, bad habits are going to do the opposite and will place you into rigid and negative behaviours. These habits, such as driving above the speed limit, smoking, and overeating, are going to make life more difficult and can damage your wellbeing and health.

The issue with habits is that we need to consciously decide which ones are good and which ones we need to kick out. The subconscious mind is not able to determine the difference between bad and good habits. It just sees that you are repeating the activity over and over so it turns it into a habit. This is why bad habits are just as hard to break as anything else. You have to retrain the brain to understand that this action is no longer a habit like it once was. This is hard to do and you have to think about it every day to avoid falling back into the trap. Once the mind learns that this is no longer a habit, it is easier to stay away from the chosen activity, but it does take some time and work.

How Do You Form Habits?

Forming a habit is pretty simple. The brain is going to start to recognize when you do the same activity over and over again. It will see that this is something you should know how to do and that it would be more efficient if you barely had to think about it. Over time, this action is going to become automatic because the brain has made it into an essential habit.

For the most part, the basic habits that you employ have been in your life since you were born. Your parents would have passed on a lot of their habits to you during your formative years. Many children will model the behaviors that they see from observing the actions of others around them. In addition, the education, experiences, and personality of the person will determine what habits they have.

It is possible to make changes to your habits. The brain is always looking for a new habit because it is looking for patterns in life. Patterns make things easier, something that is hard to come by when the world is always so confusing. When you redo an action over again, the pathways to the brain for that action will start to get wider and stronger, an action by the brain that helps it to understand that this is something important.

So how can you use this to your advantage? If you would like to drop an old, bad habit, you need to make sure that you are doing it in the right way. This will be discussed a bit later in the guidebook, but don't just try to stop the old habit. The brain likes to have patterns and efficiency to keep things in order. It is going to have trouble getting rid of the old habit without something as a replacement. Bad habits are like a comfortable bed, easy to get into but hard to get out of.

Let's say you want to stop your bad habit of overeating. Instead of trying to go on a diet, find a new habit that will help you to get over it. A good example is to start working out. Any time you have a craving for something and aren't feeling hungry, don't go and grab a candy bar or another plate of food. Instead, do a quick run around the block or fifty jumping jacks. This is going to help you to get healthier, eat less, and form some good habits with your brain to replace the bad ones.

Habits are all around you. If you took the time to look at all the actions that you are able to do in the day without even thinking about it, you would be amazed. These habits are meant to make life easier, which is sometimes why it is so hard to break them. But with the right mindset and some hard work, you can get everything in order and start to develop some new habits that are good for you!

Chapter 3 How to Enrich Your Life With Good Habits

As noted above, your thinking process and your outlook on life can change your entire path to success. Sometimes when you find yourself in the process of creating new habits, you might often find yourself on a mental block. In order to find success, and overcome these mental blocks you simply need to address the way you think. Focus on the positives and always look for ways to find new path or solutions. A great technique to find a solution to any of your problems is explained below.

The "technique of the ten solutions" is a great way to get out of a rut of thinking and make great progress on new habits. With this technique, you address a problem you have by coming up with ten possible solutions. Consider this example. Let's say you want to get a new car but don't have the money to do it. In order to get the funds for one, you can do the following ten things:

1. Get a part-time job and put that money aside toward the new car

2. Get a loan from a bank

3. Find a family member who can loan you the money

4. Cut out one unnecessary expense that you have monthly. Put that money away toward the purchase of the car

5. Sell furniture that you do not need in order to buy a car

6. Learn a trade (at the Library) and begin making projects to sell to save money

7. Find a family member that will give you a car and allow you to work off the cost

8. Have a garage sale of used clothes and items in your home. Put money toward a new vehicle

9. Offer to do odd jobs for money for the older people in your neighborhood

10. Advertise a particular skill you have and a rate you prefer to be paid (dog walker, wood carver, etc...)

Do the previous exercise every time you find yourself stuck in a problem and you will begin to see how good answers and ideas come to you. You can use this technique anytime you find yourself stuck on a way to approach and accomplish a new goal or habit.

Chapter 4 Tips to Stick Your Habits

Having some trouble getting started on your journey to making good habits? Don't sweat it! These things take time and they are going to be difficult. This is how our body works. To be efficient, you need to do the same things every day and when you try to change up the way that you act, your body and brain are going to resist. That doesn't mean you are going to fail. It simply means that you need a bit more motivation, practice, and time to make it all work for you. If you are struggling, follow some of these easy tips to get you started:

- Do it for 30 days—when you want to get started on a new habit or to drop an old one, just commit to 30 days. This is just a few weeks. While it might be some of the hardest weeks you have every dealt with, you will be able to get through all of this and see some results. If you can make it through the few weeks, you will see such an improvement in your life. Plus, your brain will start to see this new activity as a habit and you will just get up and do it without thinking.

- Stick with it each day—you must stay consistent if you would like to get this habit to stick. For example, if you plan to start an exercise program, you need to try and make it to the gym each day for the first month. This might seem like overkill, but in the beginning you are teaching your body that the gym is important and that you need to go. You can loosen this up a bit later on once you have made it a habit. But only going to work out three days a week makes it take longer to become a habit.

- Start with something simple—never try to change your life overnight. This is just not going to work. It is going to leave you frustrated and make failing even easier than before. Start out with something simple or set up milestones to help meet your goal.

- Set a reminder—you will find that after two weeks, it becomes easier to forget about your goals. Don't let this happen otherwise you will begin to slip back into some of your old habits. Find a way to place reminders about the habit all around you so that you don't miss out on any days. Missing out on the activity is going to defeat all your hard work to start with.

- Find a buddy—if you can find someone who will do the activity with you, this is going to make things so much easier. You will have someone who pushes you and is a motivating factor along for the whole ride. You have to hold yourself accountable when another person is present, making it harder to just give up or go back to the bad habits that you had before.

- Find a trigger—this is basically some ritual that you are going to use right before you perform the new habit. An example of this is when you are trying to quit smoking. Whenever you feel like you want to have a cigarette, you could start snapping your fingers instead. If you plan on getting up earlier in the morning, you might want to implement the same rituals into the morning to make this process easier as your body gets used to the new routine.

- It's ok to be imperfect—it is fine to fail once or twice along the way. Giving up an old habit is tough. You don't want to beat yourself up too much over all this or you may feel like it is all hopeless. Realize that mistakes are going to happen and that these mistakes are not the end of the world. This takes off some of the pressure and makes it easier to dust yourself off and get back to work after you fall.

- Get rid of the temptation—try to change your environment as much as possible so that you aren't being tempted by the things that will get you back onto your old habits. You can get rid of those cigarettes if you want to stop smoking, cancel the cable if you want to be more active and stop watching TV, or get rid of the bad foods if you are on a diet. When you get rid of the temptations, it is much easier for you to stick with your plans and see some results. While you are at this, make sure to find something that will stand in as comfort when you are done. If TV or cigarettes were a way to calm you down, it is going to be almost impossible to calm down without them during this 30 days. Consider meditation, reading, or some type of exercise to keep yourself relaxed and away from the bad habit.

- Do it as an experiment—worried about failing when you try out this process? Take a different approach. Do everything that you would need to in order to get rid of your bad habit or add in a new one for the 30 days. Don't judge yourself during this time. Just see this as an experiment to determine how well you can do the process. It is not possible to fail when you are doing an experiment, so you won't feel so terrible when things don't go your way one hundred percent. And at the end, it is likely that you have developed the new habit that you want.

- Do it because you want to—when forming a new habit, do not concentrate on the reasons that you should do the habit or all of the other habits that you should be working on. This is not going to make you feel good about yourself. These are just going to be full of empty resolutions that will never become fulfilled because you don't care all that much, but will still make you feel bad because of the guilt. Rather than letting this get to you, find a habit that you would like to implement into your life, one that you are passionate about, and work towards that.

- Getting a good habit to stick can be a challenge. You are going to need to work hard to see results and it will not happen overnight. But when you try out some of these tips and stick with your resolutions, you will soon see that good habit become a part of your regular routine without having to think about it.

Chapter 5 Build Self-Love & Positivity

Many of us don't love ourselves quite enough.

We claim we're doing fine, we work towards being kinder and more forgiving of ourselves and of our actions. But do we truly *love* ourselves?

It seems altogether too narcissistic to feel 'self-love' and it's kind of embarrassing too. We dodge the subject, thinking that we're not deserving enough of our own love, or thinking that we are only permitted to love those around us and not ourselves.

But this is part of the problem we have with our happiness and sense of fulfillment. Inject a little self-love and positivity into your life by fostering some healthy habits, and you can achieve so much more than you have ever imagined.

Then let's think about what happens when you *don't* love yourself.

When You Don't Love Yourself Enough

Consider that inner voice that silently passes comment on your behavior and your attitude, endlessly attempting to sabotage your success and your happiness. It drums it into your head that you are somehow substandard, unlovable, a failure, a fraud and any other negative adjective you can think of. It tells you that your worst-case scenario will probably come true and will make a mountain out of a molehill. Now what kind of life is this? Living as a victim of that inner voice that has no basis in truth whatsoever and only serves to bring you down.

You might think that there can be no escape from this horrible voice and that it's just how you were made, but I have to tell you right now that you are wrong. Completely wrong.

The difference between the positive people who love themselves and the negative who dislike their own existence comes down to only one thing: how closely they listen to that inner voice of negativity.

The positive ones know the truth and brush away the lies this voice might whisper, and the negative ones avidly listen to every word and take them as law, limiting themselves and their behavior in the process.

How to Find Your Self-Love

I don't want you to be one of these people who never attain their dreams due to the iron-like grip of this voice. Nothing in your life will ever improve if you continue to let it dominate your life.

The journey towards fostering self-love and positivity is easier said than done, but with the following few tips, you'll be surprised just how easily it comes.

1) Every day tell yourself you are brilliant and worthy of all that the world has to offer. Look into the mirror, gaze into your eyes and remind yourself how brilliant you really are.

2) Take your time to reflect on your life and the world around you. Through reflection we can learn to identify our negative habits and develop more positive ones.

3) Don't compare yourself to others. You are unique. You are beautiful. There is no one like you in the world, and that is amazing.

4) Develop a thicker skin and don't take the actions of others too personally. It's probably not about you at all, but instead their mood or their own personal circumstances that you're not aware of.

5) Banish that victim mentality. You are responsible for your actions, no one else. Nor are you to blame for the actions of others.

Practice these steps and you will be astonished at how much better you feel and just how quickly you can train your brain into loving yourself more and more each day.

Chapter 6 How to Change Your Thinking From Negative to Positive

Sometimes the best way to make a change in your habits is to change the way that you think about life. If you are a pessimist and see everything as bad or harmful to your wellbeing, you are less likely to be willing to make the changes needed to have good habits. On the other hand, those who are optimists and better able to see the good in life will see that it is easier to get these good habits. This chapter is going to take some time to talk about how the way you view the world is going to affect your habits.

The Law of Attraction

The first thing that we will discuss is the law of attraction. This is going to have a huge influence on the things that are going to come into your life. The idea behind the law of attraction is that what you think about and focus on are going to influence the things that come into your life. The universe is just going to give you back the energy that you are giving out. It does not matter if that energy is good or bad; the universe is going to focus on the energy. It is going to assume that the energy you are sending out is exactly what you want.

For example, if you are dealing with a lot of negative things in your life, such as trouble with your job, a lot of debt, and other things that you wish would go away, it is because these are the things that you focus your attention on. If you continue to focus on all the bad things that are going on in your life, more of this bad luck is going to come back to you.

On the other hand, if you are having a lot of good things in your life, it is because you focus on the good things. You are thankful for the different opportunities that you have been given in life. You enjoy being with friends and family and can take the time to enjoy the small things. Because you are able to think about all the good in your life, the universe is going to send more back to you.

So what this means is that when you want to make a change in the way life is working around you, you need to be able to change the way that you think about life. If you are tired of all the bad things in your life, start to think about how you would like it all to change. What good things can come in your life that would make you happy?

What good habits would make all of the difference? When you concentrate your efforts on these, you will find that the good things will start to head your way and your life gets so much better.

You can use the law of attraction to your benefit. Instead of being upset that the good habits aren't coming your way, instead consider what is going to happen when you finally meet your goals. This makes it easier to get to the end result and you are going to love how good you feel when you are done.

How to Change Your Thinking

Before you are able to change your habits to good ones, you need to be able to change the way that you think about things. Many people spend their time talking and thinking things that are negative. They think they are going to fail from the beginning and then they are upset when they do end up failing. They don't see life in a positive way and then they are only attracting more negative things into their lives.

There is a better way to go about all of this. Learning how to take that negative thinking and turn it into more positive thinking can go a long way. You will be amazed at how much better things are in your life when you think in a positive way, just because of the law of attraction. So when you are ready, here are some of the steps that you can take in order to change the way you think about life.

Negative Self Talk is Bad

Those words and thoughts that you have in your head are considered self-talk. They are the little voice inside your head that is looking at the way that you interact and perform out in the world. For those who have a lot of negative self-talk, you will find that your levels of self-esteem are going way down, making it harder to change to the good habits that you are looking for.

Instead of dealing with the negative self talk, it is important to learn how to change it to positive. When you want to berate yourself for doing poorly on a test or on something else, stop right away. Focus on the things that you did right. Did you answer some of the harder questions on the test that others missed? Did you get out and try a new workout that week, even though you weren't able to keep count and keep up with the others?

There is always something that you do well when you perform a task. Ignore all of the things that went wrong, there are plenty of those, and then focus on just the things that you did well, there is always at least one or two of these in each situation. Before long, you will start to feel better and the positive thoughts in your head begin to sound much better.

Use Humor

If you aren't able to see the humor in life around you or to have some fun, you will find that it is impossible to be positive all of the time. Always be open to some humor and laughter. This doesn't mean that you have to sit around laughing all of the time, but just see that there is the potential for some humor in all situations. This can take away some of the stress that you are feeling and can help to make the outlook on the situation so much better.

Optimism is Your Friend

Try to think in a positive way about everything that is going on in life around you. Even when something is not going the way that you want, figure that things are only going to get better or find a way to make them work for you. Those who are optimists are more likely to follow good habits and have a more positive life because they refuse to let the bad and negative thoughts get to them.

If you are having a lot of trouble getting used to a good habit, you are more likely to be a pessimist. These people are extra hard on themselves and might be grumbling a lot about nothing. You should learn how to see the good in all situations and try to be an optimist about the future; this will help you see the results so much easier.

Keep on Going

You should never try to turn off the positive thinking. This is not something that you can turn on and off whenever you need. Even those who are born happy and optimistic find that it is difficult to think in a positive way all of the time. You need to find a way to stick with this kind of thinking for the long term, no matter how bleak things are going to get. While there are going to be times when you think some negative thoughts, you can work to minimize these thoughts and get them turned around before they start to take over your whole life.

Find some friends

Before you start to try and change the way that you think about life, you should make sure to enlist some of your friends to help you along the way. You can have them there to be your cheerleaders to encourage you along the way to success. If possible, you should ask some friends or family members to help you out with getting some positive thoughts. You can all work together in order to have better thoughts and see an improvement in the way that you view life.

Positive thinking can make a huge difference in the way that you view your whole world. Once you are able to see things in a more positive light, it is easier to let go of all the bad habits that are holding you back and instead work on the good habits that you are looking for. This is going to take some time, but it is well worth the work to make things easier when it comes to your habits.

Chapter 7   Develop a Morning Routine

Too many of us rush around from the very moment we open our eyes. The alarm pulls us from our dreams and we get caught up in a whirlwind of rushed preparations for the day, chaos and confusion and stress, and spend far too much time hunting the car keys, choosing what to wear, wrestling the kids into appropriate clothing or asking them to brush their teeth. It's making me feel frazzled just thinking about it!

Now imagine you could start your day in a whole different way. Imagine you could wake slowly, welcome the morning with open arms and gently blow the cobwebs of sleep away from your body. Imagine a calm, soothing, peaceful start to the day. Sounds awesome, doesn't it?

You can make this dream become a reality by changing the way you look at your morning and starting some new healthy habits that will take your mood from stressed to soothed.

Here's what you need to do:

- Collect and prepare everything that you'll need for your day the night before
- Wake at least ten minutes earlier and give yourself extra time to clear your mind and gather your thoughts before you launch out of bed
- Use this time to reflect and ask yourself what you are grateful for, to encourage a positive mindset *(see 'Habit 26' for more detail)*
- Start the day right by making the time to enjoy a short yoga session, a series of stretches, positive affirmations or meditation
- Mentally plan out your day while you are in the shower and uninterrupted - focus on your priorities first
- Make time to enjoy a healthy and wholesome breakfast, such as oatmeal with fresh berries, to fuel you for the day ahead.

Implementing a 'slow' morning routine rather than a tensed, stressed one will help you and your family start the day with a smile and an air of positivity.

Chapter 8   How to Make the Decision to Take Action

Sometimes the best way to make sure that you are changing your bad habits for good habits is to think about the decisions that you are making. Those with bad habits are going to make decisions in a different way than those who have good habits. This chapter is going to take a look at the two different ways to help determine how they each work and which one is the best for you.

Decisions of Those with Bad Habits

First, we will take a look at the decision making process of those with bad habits. The first thing that this group will look at is their feelings. They will think about how they are feeling at the moment. Are they tired and want to just relax in front of a good movie or their favorite show. Are they having some cravings for some other weakness and just want to give in. They are looking at their feelings in the now and not caring about what will happen later.

Next, the people in this group are going to think about the action that they should be doing. For instance, they know they should not be watching TV for that long, but the feeling of comfort is just too strong that they end up doing nothing and it goes on for days, even weeks or more, because that's the habits they are building, the habits of cancelling what they should be doing already. There is a quote by Karen Lamb that says, "A year from now you will wish you had started Today." So why waste time when you know you should be acting on it already. Again, this is because most people like being in their comfort zone. The comfort zone is a beautiful place but nothing ever grows there. They will stay in the same place, they will never improve. or for example they will decide that the craving for the cigarette is just too strong, they will say I will stop Monday or another day or just one last cigarette, but they know deep down this is just an excuse to make themselves feel better. No matter what the stimulus is all about, they will feel that their need is strong and they won't care as much about the decision. In most cases, they are going to act on the feelings that they are having.

By this point, they are finally starting to make the decision that they had settled on in the beginning. They remember that they were supposed to stop smoking and shouldn't have had that cigarette because it would ruin all of their hard work and motivation. Of course, by this point, they have already done the action so it is too late. They are going to feel bad and like they are failures, but it is too late to do anything about it. This becomes a vicious cycle because the person will keep acting on their initial feelings.

Decisions of Those with Good Habits

The way that a person with good habits thinks about an action is going to be a bit different. They are going to first keep their decision in mind. Instead of this being at the very end of the discussion, it is going to be at the beginning. They remember the promise to eat healthy and to stick with the diet or work on their business and be productive. They know that they are going to feel so much better if they avoid all things that are bad for them and not procrastinate on their goals. They always have this decision in mind and won't let anything else get in their way.

Now, with the decision in mind, they are going to act. They will work on the tasks they have whether they feel like it or not. If the task is too boring they can choose to get a coffee break to get some boost to get going with the task. They will pick an action that works with the situation and that keeps them from giving in to their craving of watching TV instead of getting the work done for example and do something that would ruin their plans.

Finally, at this point the person with good habits is going to think about their feelings. They are going to have overlooked their feelings of cravings to do something good for themselves. Now they can enjoy the feelings that are to come next. if they are on a diet, they will feel good that they got in a fantastic workout instead of eating too much. They are going to feel good for their dedication and for all the good exercise that they were able to get done.

So when you want to change up some of your habits and make them into good habits, remember to think based on the second example. This will make it much easier to see results.

Chapter 9   How to Stay Fit Without the GYM

How did people stay fit before fitness equipment? Truthfully, before fitness equipment was invented, people were actually in much better shape. But the equipment itself isn't at fault. It's a byproduct of a society that has become too busy, and possibly too lazy, to focus on health.

Hitting the gym isn't a bad thing. You can definitely achieve your fitness goals there. The point is simply that it is not necessary.

There are plenty of other ways to get fit. We'll cover some ideas to get you started, but first, a word on forming new habits.

Forming an Exercise Habit

It's great to have goals, but you don't have to jump in with both feet and run a marathon. Figure out your exercise comfort zone, and then kick that up a notch. This will be your starting point. But in order for exercise to become part of your life moving forward, it must become a habit.

To form a new habit, you don't need to do the same workout every day. And thank goodness – because that's not even recommended for optimal fat loss. All you have to do is create a routine.

If you plan to work out every morning, part of your routine may be laying out your clothes the night before. Then, you get up and pop in a yoga DVD or grab the dog's leash and go for a brisk walk. When you're in the habit of working out at the same time each day, not only are you more likely to actually get the workout done, but you're also more likely to keep it going over time.

Make exercise fun!

When exercise is a chore, it's going to be treated as such. But did you know that exercise can actually be something you look forward to doing? It's really true! Check out these fun ideas for getting pumped about exercise:

Dance the fat away – Dance is exercise too! As long as you're moving your body, you're burning calories. You can start with something low-intensity like ballroom dancing and work your way up to a high-intensity Zumba class.

Play a sport – When we were kids, it was so much easier to keep the fat off because we were always moving. There's nothing to say that adults can't do the same. Even if you aren't the athletic type, there's likely a sport out there that is suited for you. Consider taking tennis lessons or joining a softball or sand volleyball team. You may even be able to find kickball in your local area. Do a little digging; you may be surprised at the fun stuff you can find!

Ride a bike – Do you remember how much fun it was to ride around the neighborhood as a kid? Well, you can feel the wind in your hair again while burning fat.

Find an exercise buddy – Exercise is always more fun with friends, so find someone whose goals are in line with your own and make plans to exercise together. First, figure out how you'll exercise. Feel free to choose one of the fun activities suggested in this book or create your own.

Consider yoga

Yoga is popular these days, but it can also be a great entry-level exercise program. It is generally a low-impact activity, so it won't be harsh on your body. Just be sure to find a beginner's class if you don't have any prior experience with yoga. Although it is low intensity, some of the more advanced classes can get intense and it's easy to hurt yourself by attempting yoga moves that your body is unprepared for.

Consider walking

Walking is a gentle low-impact form of exercise that almost anyone can do. It's easy, free and suitable for most people regardless of age. It doesn't require a major commitment and it may even help you get from point A to point B. So the real question should be "Why not walk?"

Walking strengthens the heart

Daily walks have been shown to reduce the risk of heart disease and stroke by lowering bad cholesterol and increasing good cholesterol and keeping blood pressure in check at the same time. Virtually any movement that raises your heart rate and gets your blood pumping is a workout for your heart. To get the most out of your daily walks, be sure to keep the pace up. Walking two or three hours a week can reduce your risk of stroke by up to thirty percent.

Walking burns calories

When you're trying to lose weight, burning more calories than you're eating is like the holy grail. In fact, experts recommend that you aim to burn about 600 calories a day more than you consume. Walking is quite possibly the easiest way to accomplish this goal. Simply put one foot in front of the other. A 143-pound person will burn 100 calories by strolling at just two miles per hour for 30 minutes. Bump it up to three miles per hour and you're burning as many as 99 calories. At a brisk four miles per hour, you'd burn 120 calories.

Walking is also an effective way to increase your muscle mass, and the more muscle you have the better your body will become at burning fat.

Walking tones your legs and butt

You can usually tell when someone has committed to walking daily because the shape of their legs becomes more defined. They have greater definition around their calves, quads, hamstrings and they also have a more lifted butt (hilly terrain helps with this part). And if you practice good posture while you're walking, you can even tone your abs and blast fat around your waist.

Before you start walking, do a posture check. Stand up straight and roll your shoulders up (towards your ears), back and then down. Think of the motion as tucking your shoulders into their proper place in your back. As you walk with this posture, your shoulders will rotate naturally to work your abdominal muscles. Just be conscious of your posture as you go along, but try not to be too rigid about it.

Power-walking tones your arms

To take your stride from a stroll to a power walk, hold your arms at a comfortable level, bent at the elbow, and swing them backwards and forwards as you walk at a brisk pace. The faster you swing your arms, the faster you'll likely walk. It may not seem like much, but this movement will tone your arms, shoulders and upper back

Chapter 10   Foods to Eat and Avoid

FOODS ALLOWED

Check out the list of nutritious and delicious food choices that should be incorporated in your daily diet to lower your cholesterol level in no time. If you make these food choices part of daily meals, in less than four weeks you'll see improvements on your cholesterol level and you'll feel healthy.

Wheat & Grains

The majority of your diet will be based on wheat and other healthy grains. These are great sources of fiber and are low in cholesterol. These are also good for the heart and lessen your chance of developing heart disease.

The mindset should be to replace any white bread, white pasta, white grain and white flour with wheat products. Remember, white is unhealthy so stick with brown or wheat-based products.

Examples are wheat bread, wheat pasta, wheat flour, quinoa, couscous and oatmeal.

Potato & Sweet Potato

These are rich in good carbohydrates, low in calories, and filling which make them ideal as side dishes in meals.

Low-Fat Dairy Products

Low-fat milk, cheese, and yogurt are your new refrigerator essentials. They provide the same amount of calcium needed by the body, minus the high fat content. Ideally, a person must consume 2-3 portions of low-fat dairy products every day.

Examples are low-fat milk, soymilk, skimmed milk, Greek yogurt, unflavored yogurt, yogurt ice cream, cottage, curd and other low-fat cheeses.

Fruits & Vegetables

These two are the essentials in a low-cholesterol diet. Add fruits and vegetables in your breakfast, lunch, dinner and snacks. Instead of reaching for junk foods, like a bag of potato chips, munch on carrot sticks.

These are rich in fiber, anti-oxidants and vitamins that benefit the body. These aid in flushing out cholesterol stuck in the body.

Legumes

Examples of legumes are white beans and red beans. These are filling and they contain no cholesterol. These are staple elements in a low-cholesterol diet, being substitutes for white rice, white pasta, and white bread.

Fish & Shellfish

These are good sources of Omega-3, which is good for the heart. They lower the risk of developing heart disease, plus they're a good alternative to meat products. Both fresh and canned fish can be incorporated in your weekly meals.

Examples are salmon, mahi-mahi, tilapia fillet, cream dory, crab, shrimp, and squid.

Eggs

Consume only the egg whites because yolks are high in cholesterol. When cooking eggs, use as little oil as possible. Better yet, consume hard-boiled eggs and remove the yolk.

Beverages

You may consume carbonated and caffeine based drinks, however alcohol intake should be limited. If you want to drink alcoholic beverages, choose white or red wine. These types of wine are good for the heart when taken in moderation.

Smoothie & Juicing

These are a great addition to low-cholesterol diets. A healthy juice or smoothie is made of at least 60% green leafy vegetable and 40% fruit. Also, the liquid base to be used should be either water or almond milk. Any artificial sweetener added to the juice or smoothie makes it unfit for low-cholesterol diets.

Examples of fruits and vegetables commonly used in juicing or smoothie-making are strawberries, blueberries, bananas, apples, spinach leaves, celery, and kale leaves.

Condiments and Spices

To keep your dishes flavorful, using certain condiments and dried herbs is allowed. These help keep the food appetizing and flavorful.

Examples of condiments and dried herbs to be

used in this kind of diet are Worcestershire sauce, vinegar, soy sauce, mustard, garlic powder, thyme, and rosemary.

FOODS THAT SHOULD BE AVOIDED

Below is a list of foods that should be avoided while undergoing a low-cholesterol diet. Stay away from the following food products:

White Grain & Flour

Avoid anything white when it comes to bread, pasta, and rice grains. These white ingredients contain low amounts of fiber. Therefore, these will not help in lowering your cholesterol. These ingredients are also responsible for increasing blood sugar, so it's best to use wheat products instead.

Butter

A common ingredient used in cooking and baking, known for its delicious and creamy flavor. One stick of butter contains a whopping 81% of your recommended daily allowance of cholesterol. The next time you want to put butter in your food, remember that what you're about to eat is plain cholesterol.

Egg Yolk

One egg yolk contains 180 miligrams of cholesterol. People with high cholesterol are advised to eat the egg whites only.

Shrimp

Shrimp are relatively small in size, but are loaded in cholesterol. Just 3.5 ounces of cooked shrimp provides the total recommended daily allowance of cholesterol.

Caviar

Commonly used as spread for breads and toppings for appetizers. For every 1 Tablespoon of caviar, it contains about 31 per cent of your recommended daily allowance of cholesterol. That's too high!

Fast Food

A regular burger in any fast-food chain normally contains 40-90gm of cholesterol. Preservatives and oils are added in making burger patties, chicken fingers, and fries. Plus, the oil used in their kitchens is repeatedly used, which in turn is unhealthy and often leads to cancer.

Peanut Butter

This favorite spread among many is ideal for people needing a boost of energy. However, for every 1 Tablespoon of peanut butter, there's 8 grams of fat. For a snack item, it is very rich in cholesterol.

Processed Meat

These include hotdogs, bacon, sausage and fast-food burger patties. These products are high in cholesterol because of the added oil used while processing them. Such products contain anywhere from 60-180 (or more) grams of cholesterol.

For example, a single slice of bacon contains 8-10 mg of cholesterol.

Full-Cream Dairy Products

These include full-cream milk, cheese and ice cream. These products are rich in cholesterol and sugar. For example, cream cheese tastes good on breads and baked goodies but 1 oz of it already has 27 mg of cholesterol.

Avocado

Though avocado is considered a fruit, every cup of it is equivalent to 21 grams fat and 3.1 grams saturated fat. Studies have shown that people who consumed avocado on a weekly basis had an increase in their cholesterol levels.

Coconut & Coconut Milk

A half-cup of coconut meat contains about 12 grams fat, while one-cup of coconut milk contains 57 grams fat and 51 grams of that is saturated fat. Opt for coconut water, which is healthier.

Organ Meats

These include liver, foie gras, heart and intestines. These parts of the animals are rich in cholesterol. For example, liver is responsible for producing cholesterol in the body. Therefore, eating liver is directly eating cholesterol in its purest form.

Salt & Soy Sauce

Salt, whether rock, iodized or pink form should be avoided or used sparingly when cooking. Salt and soy sauce cause water and fat retention in the body. Cholesterol stays longer in the walls of the cells when water retention happens.

Duck Meat

Though not everyone eats duck on a regular basis, a small serving of duck meat contains 100 mg of cholesterol.

Dietary Overview:

- Total fats should be no more than 25% of your total calories for the day

- Saturated fats should be less than 7% of total calories

- Polyunsaturated fats can be up to 10% of your total calories

- Mono-saturated fat can make up to 20% of your total calories

- Carbohydrates should make up roughly 50-60% of your total calories

- Proteins should equate to 15% of your total calories

- Cholesterol should be no more than 200 mg/dl per day

- Your diet should also include 2g of plant sterols per day and 10 – 25g of soluble fiber per day

Food Examples Per Day Amounts

- You should not eat more than 5 oz of lean meat, fish or meat/fish alternatives per day

- You can eat as many egg whites as you like, but not more than 2 egg yolks per week

- With low fat dairy products you can have 2 – 3 servings per day of products that have less than 1% fat

- Other fats and oils should not equate to more than 6 – 8 teaspoons per day

- You should try and eat more than 6 servings of whole grains per day

- Vegetables, 3 – 5 servings per day

- Fruits, 2 – 4 servings per day

Chapter 11   30 Day Plan to Live Healthy

Before You Start:

1. Before you start on any plan to live healthy you need to know what your own levels are – make an appointment to see your doctor and make a note of what your Cholesterol, HDL, LDL, triglyceride and total cholesterol levels are at the beginning of your program – that way you can measure your success as you move through this action plan. It is also a good idea to spend time talking to your doctor about any exercise routine and any other health complications you might have.

2. Write down all of your goals as well as the things you want to include in this action plan – this will keep you focused and on track. If you are a smoker include a date to become a non-smoker.

3. Talk to your friends and family about what you are doing and get a bit of support – this will help you to stay accountable.

4. Research some different exercise routines and mix things up a bit so you don't get bored with this extra activity.

5. Start planning some healthy meals that actually taste good.

Week One:

1. Think positively about your new lifestyle and launch into it with a bang. Think thin, think healthy and you will be what you think.

2. Make some small changes – reduce your consumption of whole milk and substitute with skim or 2% milk, or consider soy as a tasty and healthy alternative.

3. Schedule a couple of exercise sessions through the week – every second day is fine for a start.

Exercising Your Cholesterol Levels Back to Normal

According to the American Heart Association, you do not have to exercise too much, but they do recommend 30 minutes of moderate exercise a day. Moderate exercise is apparently enough to increase your HDL cholesterol levels and reduce your LDL levels. They also recommend that you use a variety of different routines or activities so that you get maximum results for minimum boredom.

Typically aerobics are supposed to be the most effective exercises for your heart. This can include things like jogging, jumping jacks, skipping or jumping rope, running, cycling, skiing, any racquet sports, basketball and baseball. While these activities will get your heart pumping, if you have not been doing any specific exercises in the past ten years or so you might be better off starting with water aerobics or swimming as this has less impact on your joints and is easier to do for the unfit among us. In some cases your high cholesterol readings might have already caused some damage to the heart itself, or the arteries around it, so don't plan to run a marathon in a week either. Get advice from your doctor as to what level of exercise is suitable for your age and fitness level. Some of the exercises you can do in the water can include:

1. Walking around the perimeter of the pool ensuring that your feet stay on the ground. Then second time round start to jog in the water instead

2. Try a form of cross country skiing in the water by moving in a zigzag motion bending your knees and straightening yourself as you go

3. Jumping jacks

4. Dancing

5. Walking has become a favorite stand-by doctors' use for people who loath the idea of exercising. Walking is also something strongly recommended by the American Heart Association because by just doing it 30 – 60 minutes a day you can reduce your cholesterol levels, reduce your chances of heart disease, stroke, diabetes; reduce your chances of getting cancer and increase your overall body health.

6. To make your walks more interesing trot down to your local shopping mall early in the morning and spend your time walking around that. Walk through local parks; a dog is always a willing companion on a walk. Beaches, suburban shopping centers, garden tours and hiking trails are all variations on the walking theme and all of them have their own fun element in them.

7. Start taking any supplements you have decided to take – include a multi-vitamin if your overall health is not at optimum levels. Also Vitamin C (1,000–4,000 mg per day); vitamin E (800 international units per day); Guggul (900 mg a day in three doses – see an Ayurvedic physician for supervision with this).

8. Reduce your red meat intake by at least 50%. Increase your fish and seafood meals to at least three times per week and watch what you are having as snacks. Include a vegetarian main meal once a week.

Change Your Mind, Change Your Life

Have you ever considered how your perception can change the way your day goes? Maybe you have noticed that on days when it is sunny that your heart seems to sing and your day flows by effortlessly, while on other rainy days everything seems to go wrong: traffic is a nightmare and you just want to get the day over and done with. Guess what? These days have nothing to do with the weather. They have to do with the way you feel about your day.

Let's go back to where it starts: when you wake up in the morning. You hear the rain on the roof and you groan to yourself. You mentally start running through all of the things you need to get done in the day and how the rain is just going to make that all the harder to get your day finished. How do you know that you will have a bad day when it is raining? Because it always happens, that's why. And what is even more amazing is that you are right every time. Gosh isn't it amazing how much the fact that it is raining when you get up in the morning can wreck your whole day?

Week Two

1. Now you should be getting serious about this. Increase your exercise routine to 4 – 5 times per week. if you are having trouble with scheduling your exercises then exercise in smaller chunks during the day and increase the number of times you do it. If you have to get up half an hour earlier and start your day with a walk – this is also useful for reducing stress levels.

2. Replace most of your snack foods with fruit such as apples, carrots and other fruits and vegetables. You will be starting to enjoy the crisp fresh taste of raw fruits and vegetables by now and when you are eating things like this every mouthful helps.

3. Work on your stress because stress can undo all of the good you are doing with your other lifestyle changes – start meditating at least fifteen minutes a day or do yoga. Start letting go and saying "no" to free up some time in your day.

4. Include some spices in your meals, in particular Chile peppers, garlic and onions. This combination will help grab your cholesterol and flush it straight out of your system.

Week Three

1. If you have not tried Green Tea yet then use this to boost your cholesterol lowering efforts this week. You could also try chai tea which is nuttier than green teas but just as good. If you are not sure you will like the taste then try them out at a café first (Chapter Five: Yes to Tea and Coffee).

2. Increase your use of Soy products – use soy milk in your beverages and on your cereals. Try soy burgers as a main meal with salad.

3. You should be taking 200mg of selenium per day by this stage especially if you are going to get your levels checked next week – you may already be taking it in your multi-vitamin tablets so check those first. How many times have you said "no" this week – make sure that you are not overloading your daily schedules and that your stress levels are nice and low.

4. If your stress goes up so does your cholesterol levels; so keep things calm (Chapter Three: Stress Management).

5. Use one of the dry grains for breakfast at least a couple of times this week – that could include muffins with oat or wheat bran as the main ingredient.

Week Four

By now

- Your red meat intake should be reduced by 90%;

- Your whole milk and other whole milk dairy products should be eliminated from your diet completely;

- You should have eliminated all unhealthy snacks and fatty foods from your daily diet;

- You should be exercising for at least 30 minutes four times a week or more. and

- You should have instigated a stress management program to help keep your body balanced.

If you are doing this then you are doing well.

If you have implemented just half of these suggestions your cholesterol levels will already be lower than they were three weeks ago. At this stage pick up on any of the suggestions in weeks one to three that you have not already done and make sure you do them. Also make an appointment with your doctor – it is time to check your levels again and see how you have got on.

If you get your cholesterol levels back and they are not as normal as you would like just go back to week one and start again, implementing as many of the suggestions in the three weeks outlined as you can. If you have spent a lifetime increasing your cholesterol levels, it might take a few weeks longer than the four weeks we have outlined here but you will be feeling a lot healthier at this stage and your cholesterol levels will be well on your way to the normal levels where they should be.

Regardless of what your cholesterol levels are today – if you have done four weeks then you deserve a treat and that is the only thing you have to do on day 30 – treat yourself.

Bbecause if life isn't fun, it isn't worth living.

Ten Great Recipes to Get You Started

1. BBQ Summer Vegetables & Rice

Prep: 15 min, Marinate: 10 min, Cook: 10 min.

- 2 tsp. olive oil
- 3-1/2 Tbs. chopped onions, or chopped green onion
- 2 Tbs. balsamic vinegar
- 2 cloves garlic, crushed
- 2 tsp. Dijon mustard
- 1/8 tsp. black pepper
- 3/4 medium yellow summer squash, cut into 1/2 inch rounds
- 3/4 medium green zucchini, cut into 1/2 inch rounds
- 3/4 medium eggplant, cut into 1/2 inch rounds
- 11 ounces fresh asparagus
- 1-1/3 cups cooked rice

Place first six ingredients in a bowl and blend thoroughly to make a marinade. Add the squash, zucchini, eggplant and asparagus to the marinade. Marinate for at least 10 minutes. Place vegetables on the grill, turning regularly and brushing with extra marinade. Cook until brown on each side. Serve over cooked rice. If desired, use part of the leftover marinade as a sauce.

2. Deviled Tofu Sandwich

Prep: 10 min.

- 1/4 lb. tofu
- 2 tsp. mustard 1/2 tsp. soy sauce 1/4 tsp. turmeric
- 1/4 cup green bell pepper, minced
- 1/4 cup onion (optional), minced
- 1/4 tsp. paprika
- 8 slices white bread, toasted if desired
- 8 lettuce leaves
- 4 slices tomato

Combine first 7 ingredients in a bowl. Spread mixture on half the slices of bread. Layer with lettuce and tomato and top with remaining bread.

3.   Baked Bean and Molasses Soup

Prep: 5 min, Cook: 15 min.

- 2 tsp. olive oil
- 3/4 onion, chopped
- 2 tsp. chilli powder
- 3/4 tsp. dry mustard
- 1-2/3 cups canned stewed tomatoes, with juice
- 13 ounces canned white beans, drained, 1/3 cup mashed
- 1-3/4 Tbs. molasses
- 1-3/4 cups water

Heat oil in a heavy saucepan over medium high heat. Sauté onions about 3 minutes, stirring until softened. Stir in chilli powder and mustard and cook another minute. Add tomatoes and their juice. Stir in remaining ingredients and bring to a boil over high heat. Reduce heat to medium and simmer 8 minutes, uncovered. Break up tomatoes with the back of a spoon. Season with salt and pepper to taste.

4.   Low Cholesterol Chicken Gumbo

- 1/2 c. flour
- 1 bunch celery
- 1 lb. fresh mushrooms, thin sliced
- 1 bunch (about 6) green onion, chopped sm.
- 1 med. onion, chopped sm.
- 1 lb. lean baked chicken, cut into 1/4" cubes
- 2 tbsp. light oil
- 3 1/2 c. water 1/2 tsp. salt
- 1/4 tsp. cayenne pepper

1. Wash the celery, devein the celery with a peeling knife and then cut into thin slices.
2. Heat the oil in a large skillet, add flour and brown, stirring constantly (roux).
3. Bring water to boiling in a large pot then reduce heat. Add the roux slowly, stirring constantly.
4. Add the green onion, onion, mushrooms, celery and chicken one ingredient at a time, stirring frequently. Bring to a slow boil.
5. Add the salt and the cayenne pepper and simmer for 20 minutes. Use additional water to thin the gumbo.

5.   Low-fat, Low Cholesterol, Oatmeal Drop

Cookies

- 1 cup flour
- 1/2 tsp. baking powder
- 1/4 tsp. baking soda
- 1 tbsp. molasses 1/2 tsp. salt
- 1/2 tsp. ground cinnamon
- 3/4 c. firmly packed light brown sugar
- 1 1/2 c. Quaker Oats
- 1/2 c. corn oil
- 1 egg, beaten
- 2 tbsp. water
- 1 tsp. vanilla
- 1/2 c. raisins

In a medium-size bowl, combine flour, baking powder, salt and cinnamon. Add sugar, stir in oats. Make a well in the center; add oil, egg, water, molasses, vanilla and raisins. Stir vigorously until dry ingredients are moistened. Drop by tablespoons 2 inches apart onto an ungreased cookie sheet. Bake in a preheated 350°F oven for 13 to 15 minutes or until done. Remove cookies at once to wire rack to cool.

Yield: 2 1/2 to 3 dozen cookies.

6.   Low Cholesterol No-Guilt Brownies

- 3 oz. unsweetened chocolate, chopped
- 1 c. sugar 3/4 c. flour
- 3/4 c. low-fat cottage cheese
- 3 egg whites
- 1 tsp. salt
- Powdered sugar

Heat oven to 350 degrees. Over low heat, melt chocolate and cool slightly. In food processor, puree ingredients except chocolate and powdered sugar until smooth. Add melted chocolate and blend well. Pour into lightly buttered 8-inch square pan. Bake 20-25 minutes or until well set. Sprinkle with powdered sugar. Cut in squares.

Makes 16 squares per serving.

7.   Vegetable Casserole
servinholesterol

- 2 (10 oz.) pkgs. frozen mixed vegetables Cook vegetables according to package directions.
- 1/2 c. chopped onions
- 1 c. chopped celery
- 1 c. grated cheese (low fat Mozzarella
- 1 c. mayonnaise (no cholesterol) 1/2 c. butter (no cholesterol), melted

1 c. crushed wheat (no cholesterol) crackers. Mix first 5 ingredients and pour into a Pam-sprayed dish, topped with crushed crackers mixed with butter. Cook at 375 degrees for 25 minutes. Serves 6-8.

8.   Low Cholesterol Omelette

- 1/4 c. Egg Beater
- 1 egg white
- 1 tbsp. chopped scallion
- 1 tbsp. chopped green pepper
- 1/4 c. chopped tomato
- Garlic powder
- Black pepper

Mix all ingredients together. Cook in frying pan with Pam or "no cholesterol, no salt butter". Place on low-medium flame. Serve hot.

Conclusion

Thank you again for downloading this book!

I hope this book was able to help you learn how to build healthy Habits. Every journey begins with a single step, but as you know it takes more than that to make them stick around for the long term and positively affect the rest of your life. All you have to do is maintain these habits and enjoy the life that you really do deserve.

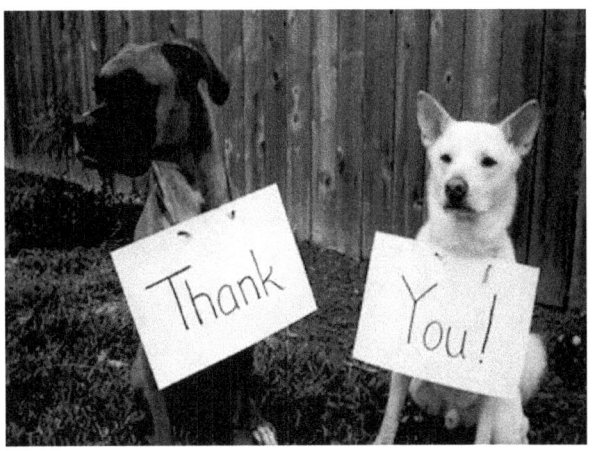

Finally, if you enjoyed this book, then I'd like to ask you for a favor, would you be kind enough to leave a review for this book on Amazon? It'd be greatly appreciated!

Click here to leave a review for this book on Amazon!

Thank you and good luck!

www.ingramcontent.com/pod-product-compliance
Lightning Source LLC
Chambersburg PA
CBHW060339290526
45793CB00003B/669